About the Authors

MICHAEL VOLIN, founder of the first yoga school in Sydney, Australia, and the foremost teacher in that country, has been teaching yoga for over a quarter of a century in Australia and in the East. He received his training in China, where he was born and brought up, and from Indian and Tibetan teachers. He was associated with Indra Devi's yoga school in Shanghai, succeeding her as director of the school when she left for the United States.

NANCY PHELAN is a writer and photographer who has published a novel and two travel books. She has been a serious student of yoga for some years and was trained as a teacher by Michael Volin. Eight other books on yoga have been co-authored by Miss Phelan and Mr. Volin.

MICHAEL VOLIN & NANCY PHELAN

Yoga for Beauty

BELL PUBLISHING COMPANY · NEW YORK

This edition published by Bell Publishing Company, Inc.,
a division of Crown Publishers, Inc.,
by arrangement with Arc Books, Inc.
A B C D E F G H

Contents

Illustrations

How to use this book

This is a practical book designed for those who would like to follow the yoga teaching of 'bringing the body to the highest state of development and maintaining it all through life'.

Yoga is not limited to physical practices; it is a profound philosophy of complete development, physical, mental and spiritual; but since training includes methods for attaining bodily perfection and prolonging the creative part of life, its connection with physical beauty is obvious.

From the 84 traditional *asanas* and countless exercises we have selected the most effective for these purposes, grouping them under the headings of *Beauty of Face* and *Beauty of Body*. Since the yoga conception of beauty is not limited to flesh and blood there is also a section on Inner Beauty.

Having decided which part of face or figure most needs improvement, check carefully through the detailed list of Contents to find the technique you require.

Regular practice and belief in the method are necessary for success. Books are not magic talismans; they cannot bring results by standing on your bookshelf – only if their instructions are understood and carried out.

Though these ancient methods have proved their efficiency they promise no over-night miracles. Progress may sometimes be slow, but it is steady and far-reaching, and benefits last as long as practice is maintained.

The exercises — as distinct from *asanas* — included here will not be found in such classical treatises as the *Hatha yoga Pradipika, Siva Samhita,* etc. Some of them ase practices of *avatara yoga,* whose teachings are, to a certain extent, concerned with conditioning and preserving the body.

Sydney   MICHAEL VOLIN
Australia   NANCY PHELAN

I

Yoga and Beauty

*'Be with me, beauty, for the fire is dying'**

This lovely line, which could express the longing of most men and women faced with time's threat to youth and physical beauty, is moving, graceful, melodious. It is also, when thus interpreted, completely negative according to yoga teaching.

The follower of yoga does not plead, 'Stay with me, beauty!' He says, 'Beauty, I shall retain you!' He does not passively let the fire die; he sets about building it up, keeping it alight long after it would have flickered out. He does not sit, sadly sighing – however poetically – about the inevitability of passing loveliness; he analyses why it is passing and works out what he can do to stop it.

He knows that if time cannot be stopped completely, it may be slowed down to a remarkable degree.

What is the connection between yoga, a reputedly austere way of life, and human beauty, with its traditional sensuous implications? The answer lies in the yogi's attitude to his body. Based on the belief that it is the temple of the living spirit, he respects it, reverences it, strives to bring it to near-perfection, mentally and physically, not only seeking to attain beauty but to retain it as

* The poet is addressing beauty in the abstract.

long as possible. In secluded *ashrams* and monasteries, certain orders of Buddhist monks practising *avatara yoga* spend hours oiling their skin, smoothing the soles of their feet with pumice stone, practising physical and mental techniques to beautify and preserve their bodies, not as a matter of vanity but out of reverence for the God who gave them these bodies. This is the first step on the path of achieving final union of the individual soul with the soul of the universe, of the individual mind with the mind of the universe . . . the ultimate goal of yoga.

In the past, certain western philosophers taught that such union or liberation came through mortification of the flesh. Even today there are followers of different sects, in east and west, living unkempt, unwashed, with matted hair and beards, smearing themselves with ashes, with cow dung; but the true yogi respects his body and cares for it to the best of his ability.

We in the West have been taught that our natural love of, joy in human beauty is faintly wrong, leading to vanity, idolatory, temptation. Puritanical phases of our history bred an unnatural shame, an impossible suggestion that man was all soul, that the flesh was corrupt, to be subjugated. Clothing was designed to conceal and smother; many parts of the body must not be mentioned; natural functions were considered shocking.

Though we have shaken off most of these hypocricies, we are still often slightly ashamed of paying too much attention to our appearance, even consider it slightly decadent. Yet we are all in love with physical beauty. In its crudest form this shows in pretty girls on magazine covers, in beauty contests . . . childish, perhaps, but nonethe-less a groping, clumsy expression of our longing for, love of human beauty.

It is generally accepted that human beauty is based on wholesomeness, naturalness, cleanliness, health; but it is not only a matter of flesh and bones; there must be personality, strength of character, spiritual awareness. The yoga ideal is inner beauty in a cared-for shell.

Classical features are given only to a few and cannot be acquired, but a well-developed, supple and agile body, smooth skin, graceful movements, serenity and beauty of expression ... a combination of physical and inner strength ... may be developed through yoga and retained for many years; should, in fact, improve with time, for true beauty is not just a matter of preserving a youthful appearance; it is a graceful adaptation to ageing at each phase of life.

Avatara yoga

This is not the place to discuss the spiritual aspects of this branch of yoga, which is associated with the laws of re-incarnation and embraces many techniques for delaying physical ageing. An *avatara* has been defined as 'One who has a combination of three elements in his being: an inspiring divinity; a highly evolved intermediate nature or soul ... the channel of that inspiring divinity; and a pure clean physical body.' This might be interpreted as a celestial being manifesting through the ageless body of a fully liberated soul.

Fundamentally based on principles of *hatha* yoga, *avatara* practices include many physical and mental techniques never yet described to the western world. Most of the preliminary methods are logical and extremely up-to-day ways of reaching the peak of physical perfection. They are passed on by mouth to ear, from teacher to disciple, in the remote *ashrams* of India, the monasteries of Tibet and China. They are closely guarded, for it is held that only the 'awakened' may appreciate the purpose behind them; and in the austere spiritual climate of these countries there are few capable of accepting the doctrine that 'there is no flower, beast or star' as beautiful as the human form.

It is believed that physical discipline and training could lead to the *avatara* state; that final spiritual enlightenment is achieved after a certain stage in the physical conquest of time, when the body becomes the vessel of the 'intermediate nature or soul.' This parallels the teaching of hatha yoga, in which physical perfection leads to victory of the spirit.

Why the body ages

Time, in the sense of ageing, is usually considered the great enemy of physical beauty; yet it is not the only destroyer. Combined ignorance, apathy, neglect year after year ... incorrect breathing; tension; chronic exhaustion; inadequate sleep; wrong diet; lack of exercise; constipation; over-exposure to weather; lack of mental interests ... all help disfigure face and body, contribute to premature ageing.

The three most powerful enemies are the *pull of central gravity, decreasing circulation in face and head, and loss of vital energy,* so frequently mentioned in this book. As the body grows older it becomes increasingly susceptible to these influences. They work together. A decline in vital energy assists the forces of central gravity; central gravity helps slow down circulation. Yoga training includes methods for combating this. There are also exercises or *asanas* for muscles, joints, spine, internal organs, nervous system, glands, circulation, and general practice could help to restore a tired and ageing body,* prolonging the best years of life in every sense. Constructive concentration and mental exercises are also included in training.

Loss of vital energy

This, perhaps, is the most serious of all, for when vital energy declines the body has lost its virtue. Life no longer seems worth living, nothing has interest, purpose, meaning. How often do we hear the words . . . 'I seem to have lost interest . . .' 'I can't be bothered any more . . .' 'I don't have the energy I used to . . .' 'I can't make the effort . . .' These unfortunates have lost their vital energy through ignorance or squandered it in the belief that they can go on for ever without paying the cost.

> 'My candle burns at both ends;
> It will not last the night;
> But – ah, my foes, and oh, my friends –
> It gives a lovely light!'

The sense of reckless gaiety is touching if the speaker drops down dead when night and candle are finished. Unfortunately this does not always happen. The devil-may-care youth goes on living, old, sick, miserable, neurotic, a burden to self and others.

* It is taught that with each new *asana* mastered the student experiences a rebirth; that in 9 months the entire body could be thus 'reborn.'

Force of central gravity

Space-flights have brought the subject of central gravity into general prominence, but to a large extent we in the west do not realize that the force holding us to the earth is also pulling us down physically, in a destructive sense.

Though the cause may not be recognized, the effects of this downward pull are familiar to us all. Sagging muscles and tissues, 'dropped' (displaced) organs, fallen arches, increasing tiredness, desire to sit or lie rather than stand are outward signs of diminishing resistance.

Yoga's remedy is simple and logical: the body is turned upside-down. The pull is thus reversed; tissues, muscles, organs that were being dragged down are now drawn the opposite way, and restored to original positions.

Decreasing circulation

At the same time, the inverted position enables the blood to flow to face and head. Some poses actually direct it there, to feed starved facial tissues. The whole system benefits; glands, organs, nerve roots receive extra supplies of arterial blood to revitalize and increase their efficiency.

Prana

The yogi sees himself as an extension of his natural surroundings; a manifestation of the life force animating all creation. He knows how to draw upon this life force for his needs, taking vital energy from the elements.

Life force is known in Sanscrit as *prana*. The main medium of intake is breathing.* (The correct method of breathing,

* The energy of sunlight, water and 'Mother Earth' is also converted to individual energy by the same process.

with recharging and pacifying breathing cycles are given in the Appendix.) As the complete yoga breath increases the volume of air inhaled, the amount of *prana* is also increased. Stale air is exhaled from the lungs but the *prana* or vital energy is directed through the body for invigorating and healing, or stored in the solar plexus as a reserve. When people say, 'He has used up all his reserve' they are speaking, no doubt unconsciously, of *prana* – vital energy.

Prana holds the body together. If supplies are not constantly replenished the whole structure crumbles. When the system is kept recharged, vitality is high; health, appearance, joy in living are at their maximum.

What is *prana?* Though its results are visible, tangible, undeniable, it cannot be seen. No one has yet bottled it, produced a synthetic laboratory-tested substitute; some find it hard to accept. If an everyday parallel must be given, it could be compared to Vitamin D in sunlight.

Prana has been described as food for the nerves. While they are soothed and restored by increased intake of life force, tension is relaxed through the slowing-down of the breath. Nervous tension destroys beauty, brings a harassed expression, awkward movements, ugly posture and chronic disturbances of digestion and glands, which also affect appearance. Correct breathing purifies the bloodstream and improves circulation in all parts of the body. Breath control is the medium by which the mind is pacified, leading to serenity of expression.

Glands

The endocrinal glands have a far-reaching influence on body, mind and attitude to life. Yoga training includes

numerous postures which benefit the glands directly, in-
directly, or both. The headstand directly stimulates the
pituitary, pineal (and thyroid), and since these are key
glands, all other glands in the system are also affected.
The shoulderstand directly regulates the thyroid, also
a key gland. *Asanas* which put pressure on the small of
the back stimulate the adrenal glands; poses in which
the lower abdomen is pressed, tone up the ovaries; certain
balancing and sitting poses affect the sex glands in men;
the balancing shoulderstand benefits the pineal gland.

Good health, optimistic and relaxed attitude to life
depend greatly on the harmonious working of the endocrinal system. 'We are just as young as our glands.' To this
might be added – 'And, to a certain extent, as beautiful
as our glands are young.'

2

Beauty of Face

All that has been said in Chapter I, on the causes of ageing, applies particularly to the face, which is not only more exposed, but reflects the personality. Neglect, ignorance, lack of inner resources, loss of vital energy, gravity forces, decreasing circulation help to dull eyes and skin, encourage shadows, sagging muscles and wrinkles.

No reasonable person expects to retain an unlined face into extreme old age, but neither do they wish to age prematurely. The happy medium is maturity, with, if need be, its lines of character, combined with firm muscles and fresh skin.

Lines and Wrinkles

Though in general, the words *lines* and *wrinkles* are given the same meaning, there is a great difference. *Wrinkles*, an actual crumpling of the skin, are usually identified with withering, neglect, ageing; *lines* with character, personality, experience of life. When a famous traveller wrote that a journey without history was like an old face without its wrinkles she probably meant character lines. The actress, Anna Magnani, certainly did when she rejected her touched-up photograph, complaining that the lines so easily wiped out had taken her a lifetime to acquire. (A number of well known actors and actresses have been better looking in maturity than in youth.)

Lines. All human faces are subject to a certain amount of change. The simple processes of living, feeling, experiencing make their marks. Every time we smile, yawn, frown, the skin is creased. These little lines, at right angles to the pull of muscles, are repeated thousands of times in a life. As the face loses youthful fat and the skin its elasticity, they deepen. When muscles are flabby, tissues starved of blood, the lines may become deep ageing furrows; but if muscles are kept firm, skin fresh and healthy, lines of maturity give strength and identity to the face, enriching rather than disfiguring.

Wrinkles. Wrinkles, as distinct from character lines, are not necessarily the honourable mark of a full life. They may come from a harsh dry climate weathering a sensitive skin; too many steam baths; faulty diet; sudden loss of weight; insomnia; tension and worry; excessive dryness from thyroid deficiency; starvation of facial tissues from poor circulation.

Starvation of Tissues. Active children, constantly bending, jumping, turning themselves upside-down, have firm glowing faces; but as they grow up the pull of central gravity, lack of exercise, sedentary occupations, help to slow down circulation to the face. Facial tissues are deprived of necessary blood; gradually the glow of health subsides, till in old age the skin of the face resembles crushed tissue paper. The logical way to delay this ageing process is to supply more arterial blood to facial tissues.

In finding this solution thousands of years ago, the yogis anticipated modern scientific beauty treatment, which works on the same principle, though by different means. Where beauticians work with electrosonic equipment, yoga uses the body itself, directing the blood to the face through inverted positions; building up pressure by combined movement and retention of breath, forward-bending and swinging exercises and by raised poses.

Pull of Gravity and Loss of Vital Energy. The effects of central gravity on the body have been described. Nowhere does its constant pull show more than in the face, manifesting as sagging muscles and tissues and a generally 'tired' look. Turning the body upside down, in inverted poses, helps to neutralize this downward pull, which is also counteracted by increasing and maintaining vital energy. Complete relaxation, regular sleep, diet, in addition to correct breathing, are essential to ensuring supplies of life force.

Loss of Facial Contours. When softly-rounded cheeks 'fall in', become drawn or hollow, the contour of the face is lost. The main cause is flabby muscles, but extraction of teeth with subsequent shrinkage of gums is a common contributor. Large gaps between back and side molars should not remain, even if they do not show. Facial exercises to restore muscle tone will help improve facial outline.

Lack of Sleep. Whoever coined the phrase 'beauty sleep' showed awareness of its importance to appearance. Not only is sleep necessary for replenishing and conserving stocks of vital energy but for relaxing facial tension, resting tired muscles and reducing strain on glands and nervous system, which react on the skin.

If possible, go to bed early twice a week* . . . ideally,

* As part of rejuvenating treatment in some countries, patients are put to sleep for up to two weeks at a time.

nights that divide the week evenly, such as Wednesday and Sunday. Do not eat too large, late, or heavy an evening meal. Allow yourself to slow down before retiring. Do some deep breathing by an open window and in bed, do not read. Lie quietly, trying to relax, keeping your thoughts from disturbing or agitating subjects, not worrying if you don't sleep at once.

If you are unused to early nights you may have a little difficulty at first, but the habit may be developed.

Yoga breathing, *Savasana*, Pose of Tranquillity help overcome insomnia. (See Appendix.)

Glands and the skin. Apart from the thyroid gland, which if disordered may cause unnatural dryness, other endocrinal glands may also affect the skin in varying degrees. In the early days of ovarian removal by radium or surgery women often aged prematurely and tragically, seeming to wither up . . . a fate which modern methods seek to avoid. Exhaustion or worry, acting on the adrenal glands, appear to change temporarily the actual texture of the skin. This is sometimes remarked before and after a needed holiday or rest . . . even after a good night's sleep.

Breathing. Every part of the face – skin, eyes, teeth, hair – owes life and beauty to the bloodstream and when this is full of impurities the appearance will suffer. The simple method of yoga breathing – described in the Appendix – should be mastered and practised night and morning, out of doors or by an open window. One can train oneself to breathe correctly even in sleep, ensuring a constant supply of vitality, relaxed nerves and a purified system.

Constipation. Indigestion. The appearance is also affected by impurities from a clogged-up digestive system. Eyes become dulled, the skin sallow, blotched, spotty. Constipation may be corrected by exercise, the education of semi-voluntary muscles, by breathing, diet and occasional fasts for purification. Poor digestion may be improved by exercise, relaxation of nervous tension, diet and the use of commonsense at meals ... careful selection of food, adequate time for eating and digesting under pleasant or at least peaceful conditions.

The complexion itself will benefit by the addition of fruit and vegetable juices to the diet. One of the most important – and pleasant – of these is strawberry juice. (The beautifying properties of this fruit is now recognized by cosmeticians who include it in certain preparations.) Less palatable but also powerful complexion aids are the juices of green peppers and raw potatoes. Mix them with carrot or tomato juice if you find them too disagreeable.

A word of warning about fruit-juices – and fruit diets. If the system is acid do not take too much acid fruit. Indigestion and spots on the face may result.

Facial tension. Although occasionally the origin may be purely physical – eye strain, pain or discomfort in other parts of the body, even tight shoes – the main causes of facial tension are the constant rush against time; trying to do too much at once; noisy distracting surroundings; stress, worry, nervous strain. The most common manifestation is unconscious frowning. Next time you cross a city street, watch the passing faces. Most of them have vertical lines between the eyebrows, even very young girls.

A yoga exercise called *Releasing of Inner Light* teaches facial relaxation (page 84). To realize the ageing, distorting effects of tension, study a sleeping face. Its strange youthfulness comes ⸀ ⸀a complete relaxation.

Pacifying breathing cycles and Pose of Complete Rest (Appendix) are also necessary part of practice in learning to release tension.

Care of the skin. Cleanliness is the basis of physical beauty, but a clean face does not necessitate drastic scrubbings, nor the use of harsh soaps. Water should be neither too hot nor too cold. (Yogis believe that energy may be absorbed from water. The revitalizing effect of a shower or swim on a tired body is well-known.)

Delicate skins need protection from strong sunlight, intense cold. Alcohol, rich food, excessive eating and drinking help destroy the complexion. Though the true yoga diet – lacto-vegetarian, devoid of all stimulants – may be impractical for western life, existing diets could be modified to advantage.

A very dry skin will benefit from regular oil baths for face as well as body, or from the addition of oil to the diet – combined with orange juice or used for cooking.

Oil baths are taken after a warm bath or shower has opened the pores. The oil is warmed (not hot) then generously rubbed in and treatment concluded, if possible, with complete relaxation. Any oil may be used – the oilier the better.

If the skin is naturally thin and dry, avoid steam, or too hot, baths – Turkish or sauna. Never steam the face nor expose it directly to harsh dry winds. Prolonged over-exposure to intense heat – as on the beach – is the surest way to destroy the complexion, apart from the possibility of developing skin cancer.

Facial Expression. When all has been done to beautify and preserve the face it will still be of little real interest if it is not enlightened from within.

We all know the beautiful creature whose flawless complexion and regular features are a façade for vacuity; and the rather plain man or woman to whom everyone gravitates, who impresses by warmth and vitality rather than physical features.

We cannot all be witty or amusing, but we could be full of vitality and a communicable sense of well-being. This may manifest as good humour, a quiet warmth, personal magnetism. It often shows as an alertness of the eyes, an interest in being alive.

A negative mind produces a negative, and consequently depressing expression; a youthful, adventurous, enquiring mind shows in young eyes that rejuvenate a lined face. By contrast, if a face smoothed out by plastic surgery retains old, tired, burnt-out eyes the effect is frightening and macabre.

Over-repressive reserve results in a dead expression. Caution, often based on uncertainty, gives a closed, baffling look. Poise that stems from inner security rather than charm-school lesson; serenity; joy in life; humour; interest in people, all make a face attractive and arresting.

But the basis of all facial expression is *vital energy*, the power by which we project ourselves to those around us.

(*ii*) *Facial exercises*

Yoga training brings ability to contract and relax every muscle of the body at will, including the so-called semi-voluntary muscles and muscles of face and scalp.

All muscles deteriorate through lack of exercise, and face and scalp are rarely exercised enough. Soft foods that need little chewing, even lack of animation, encourage flabbiness – an immobile face that shows no emotion deprives its muscles of exercise. To retain or repair muscle tone, conscious exercising must replace natural spontaneous movements.

Study your face in the mirror, analysing it with detachment in an honest attempt to see where it most needs firming. The older you are, the more important to start exercising.

There are fifteen groups of muscles in scalp and face and some familiarity with them is necessary for correct practice. The diagram on page 29 shows the position of the different groups. Study it, keep it by you for reference as you practice. It will help you to understand what you are doing and to identify the muscles you are working on. It is possible by will-power and determination to learn to control each group.

Concentrate on each part of the face in turn, 'seeing' with the mind's eye the muscles beneath the skin responding to your direction.

1. Stimulating the skin of the scalp. Put the fingers on the sides of the scalp and vigorously move it up and down 6 times. Change position of the fingers, coming further forward or backward. Repeat 3–4 times till a pleasant warmth is felt.

2. Contract and relax muscles so entire scalp is moved back and forth. The movement should be felt even in the ears. (In the way children 'wiggle' their ears.)

3. Tensing and relaxing cheeks. Tense the muscles,

28

retaining tension, then relax for a few seconds. Repeat this several times. The outward appearance is of puffing the cheeks but tension of the muscles should be felt.

4. Fill the mouth with air and, as though it were a ball, methodically roll it round inside the closed mouth,

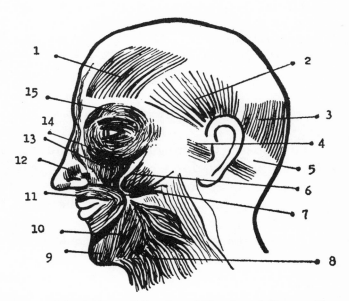

FIG. 1 The Fifteen Muscles of Head and Face. For reference in practice.

massaging cheeks and lips from within. Push the air to the right cheek, then left, under upper lip, under bottom lip.

5. Move the lower jaw from side to side, slowly, retaining extreme of each movement.

29

6. The same movement, practised rapidly and continuously.

7. Open and close the mouth like a fish gasping for breath . . . slowly, retaining each opening movement.

8. Push the lips forward, bringing them together as though blowing a kiss. The movement should be strong and definite.

9. Lift each corner of the mouth separately, then together. Make it a conscious exercise, not a grimace.

10. Turn the lips in and press them together till they disappear. Hold each movement a few seconds.

11. Bring the corners of the lips down alternately and retain for a few seconds.

12. The same movement, bringing both corners down together.

13. Combine movements, bringing the right side up, then down; left side up, then down.

14. Move both sides up and down.

15. Close the eyes, squeezing lids together, then open and blink several times.

16. Open the eyes very wide, and keep them open for 3–4 seconds.

17. Contract muscles to pull the ears up and back, separately, then together, retaining each movement for a few seconds.

18. Push the chin out, then draw it in several times. (For double chin.)

19. Imagine there is a weight on your chin which must be lifted by raising the chin and tensing muscles beneath it.

20. Tense the neck muscles vigorously, making them stand out. Retain tension for a few seconds, then relax.

21. Tense the muscles of the chin, vigorously bringing the lower lip down and inward. The movement resembles exercise No. 20, but emphasis is on chin rather than neck.

22. Smooth the lines on the forehead by contracting muscles which pull back the scalp. Retain the contraction, then relax. This is an important exercise in fighting sagging of the face and restoring firmness. (It is very similar to Exercise 17.)

23. Contract and relax the cheek muscles at the side of the nose. The movement resembles winking with right, then left eye.

24. Wrinkle the bridge of the nose.

25. Contract muscles to slightly lift the corners of the eyes. This is difficult and requires perseverence. It smooths 'crows feet' at the outer ends of the eyes.

26. Complete the cycle with *Pose of a Lion* . . . an excellent all-round exercise for the face. It is not only a beauty aid but has a powerful effect on the root of the tongue and throat.

Pose of a Lion

Sit back on the heels with the hands on the knees. Arch the back, tense the whole body and spread out the fingers, keeping them stiff and far apart. At the same time raise the head, open the eyes as wide as possible, open the mouth wide and put the tongue right out. Relax; then repeat.

Practised indoors, the eyes should be opened; outdoors – when facing the sun – they *must be kept shut.* Tilt the head so the sun's rays may enter mouth and throat.

Mind Mirror

This is an unusual mental exercise in which a form of self-hypnosis is employed. It is used in *avatara* yoga as a means of delaying ageing. Through the summoning of positive thought, of the constructive power of the mind, the student eventually frees himself – or hypnotises himself – out of fear of growing old.

The exercise is practised in the cross-legged position, after the breath has been slowed down to the rate of six heart-beats for inhalation, six for exhalation.

In the Mind Mirror you see yourself as you are now, clearly, in detail. Concentrate on evoking, establishing this likeness; then think of the future, of the years to come, and of yourself, as you are in the Mirror, never changing. Hold to the thought: *The years will pass but this face will not age.*

This technique delays further ageing. To grow younger, the yogi evokes his image of ten, twenty years before, and merges it with the present likeness, until eventually the younger completely obscures the older face. Intense concentration, will-power, patience and faith are necessary in these mental-physical exercises.

(iii) Exercises and asanas to increase circulation in the face
* *Practise exercises and asanas on a folded rug, a mat, etc., not on bare floor.*

Exercises

1. With feet slightly apart, let yourself fall forward from the waist. Upper body, head, arms should be limp as a

* Note: These exercises may also be practised for reducing and firming the waist.

rag doll . . . let yourself 'flop'. Then come up and repeat several times.

2. Let yourself 'flop' again, this time to the right side, then forward, in the same limp way. Come up and repeat several times.

3. Same movement practised to the left side.

4. With feet wider apart and arms stretched at sides, inhale, exhale as you bend forward, keeping knees straight, and grasp left ankle with right hand, pressing head to left knee. Come up and repeat on the other side.

5. With feet apart and hands on back of thighs. Inhale, exhale, bending forward, at the same time running the hands down the backs of the legs to take hold of the ankles, and trying to put the face between the knees . . . as though looking through your legs.

6. With legs apart and hands clasped on top of the head. Inhale, stretching the arms upward with the palms turned up. Exhale, coming down till clasped palms rest on the floor. Knees must be kept straight.

Cycle of asanas to increase circulation in the face

The following five *asanas* are grouped together as a cycle for their common property of accentuating the flow of blood to the face. *They are prohibited in cases of high blood-pressure.* At the end of the cycle there should be a pleasant warmth in the face, where every cell has been toned up.

       1. Head of a Cow Pose.
       2. Variation of Pose of a Child.
       3. Variation of *Yoga-mudra*.
       4. Knees-to-stomach, variation.
       5. Half-candle pose.

1. *Head of a Cow Pose*

Kneel on the floor and sit back on the heels. Correctly, the ankles should be crossed, but if this is uncomfortable, modify as above. Raise the right arm and with bent elbow behind the head, reach down the back as though to scratch between the shoulderblades. Put the left arm behind the back at the waistline and reach up until right and left hands are locked. If at first the hands cannot meet, use a handkerchief as extension.

With the hands locked, hold the pose with eyes closed and face relaxed, deeply inhaling and exhaling. Concentrate the mind on increasing circulation to facial tissues, to firming and toning up the skin. In time a warmth will be felt on the left side of the face. Conclude by exhaling and bending forward, hands still locked, till the forehead touches the floor.

Sit up, change arms and repeat.

The pose must be practised on both sides, for when the right arm is raised the left side of the face benefits, when the left arm is up it is the right side that receives extra blood. The raised elbow should show above the head. This becomes easier to achieve as muscles loosen up with practice.

2. *Pose of a Child* . . . Variation

This *asana*, popular as a pleasant relaxing position, is normally practised with arms by the sides. In this variation the position of the hands increases the flow of blood to the head.

Kneel down and sitting back on your heels, lean forward and rest the forehead on the floor. Try not to rise up at the back.

34

Clench the fists and press them together behind the back, as high up towards the shoulderblades as possible. Hold the pose, inhaling and exhaling. A warm, full sensation in the face is very quickly felt.

3. *Yoga-mudra* – Variation

This sitting pose should correctly be practised with the legs in the lotus position but if this is impossible, or inadvisable through varicose veins, sit with legs crossed.

Lock the hands behind the neck with the thumbs resting below the point of the jawbone, in the region of the jugular vein.

Inhale, exhale, then lean forward till face rests on the floor, at the same time pressing with the thumbs. With head still down, inhale again, releasing thumb pressure. Exhale as you come up.

A very powerful technique for bringing extra blood to the face.

Practice carefully.

4. *Knees-to-stomach*

A simple *asana* combined with retention of breath.

Lying on the back, inhale and draw the knees up to the stomach. Press them against the body with the hands, retaining pose and breath until you feel the whole face flushed with blood. Then release, exhale and lower the legs.

5. *Half-shoulderstand or Half-candle Pose*

Lie on your back. Bring the legs up and support your hips with your hands, elbows resting on the floor. The body is at an angle but the legs are straight. Keep the chin well away from the chest so the blood may flow freely to the face. Hold the pose, deeply inhaling and exhaling, with eyes closed and facial muscles relaxed until you feel the cheeks growing warm and full, as the blood reaches the tissues. The longer you hold the pose, the greater the benefit.

To complete, bring the legs down over the head, bending the knees and taking hold of the toes. Pull the legs out straight till the toes touch the floor; hold a couple of seconds, then let go and slowly bring arms and legs back to starting point.

The power of the mind should be brought into play during practise. While holding the pose you should try to see yourself ever young, unchangeable. *Half-shoulderstand is strictly forbidden in cases of high blood-pressure.*

Further asanas to benefit the face
Pose of a Hare

The easiest way to get into this position is from Pose of a Child. Raise the body so back and buttocks are up, with the hands on the ankles. The crown of the head, instead of the forehead, is on the floor. Hold the pose, inhaling and exhaling. Though less powerful, this is an alternative to the Headstand.

Forward-Stretching Cycle

All forward-stretching movements, sitting or standing, help improve the circulation in the face. Further variations of the following may be found on page 72 (Beauty of Body).

Sit with the right leg stretched in front and the left bent at the knee with the left foot under the right thigh. The hands rest on the knees. Inhale, exhale and bend forward until you can take hold of the right foot with the head pressed to the right knee. Come up, repeat, then practise with the left leg stretched and the right foot under the left thigh.

The effects are intensified if, after exhaling, the head is kept pressed to the knee, a further breath inhaled, retained a few seconds, then exhaled as you sit up.

Headstand. (Plate 1) This should be practised on a folded rug or blanket; also close to a wall, not in the middle of the room

Kneel down, lock your hands together and stand them on the floor, with palms facing towards you. With the elbows on the floor, lean forward and put the head inside the little enclosure made by the hands and arms. (The head should be on the floor, not on the hands, which are now locked lightly round the head.) Straighten the legs out behind you with feet on the floor and walk in towards your body. When you are close enough try to kick yourself up. As you become stronger you will be able to bring the legs up slowly and as confidence increases you could practise further away from the wall until finally you are standing unaided in the middle of the room. (Plate I).

To come down, bend the knees and bring them down, right in to the body till they actually touch the stomach; then slowly lower the legs till the feet are on the ground.

The position of the head is important. The point of contact with the floor should be approximately halfway between the hair-line and the crown of the head. The neck and back should be in one straight line. If you rest the forehead on the floor the neck will be bent back; if point of contact is too far back balance is destroyed.

Practice is the only way to master the headstand. It should never be performed after eating or drinking, or held too long. Inhale and exhale deeply and rhythmically while holding the pose. Do not attempt it if there is high blood-pressure or weak eye capillaries.

Raised Poses

These *asanas*, which are designed to preserve the body's relative strength and buoyancy, also have beautifying powers in sending extra blood to the face. They are not to be practised if there is high blood-pressure, heart disease or prolapse of the uterus.

Pose of a Bird

Squat with the knees well apart and toes together. The arms are between the legs, the hands on the floor with fingers spread out like a bird's claws. Do not keep the hands too close to the body or you may pitch over them and fall on your face. Inhale, rise up on the toes and lean forward, pressing the legs against the arms – the inner thighs against the outside of the arms – riding on your arms till your toes leave the floor. The weight is taken on the hands. Exhale as you come down.

The movement should be smooth and slow, with no jumping.

Pose of a Raven

A variation of the Bird Pose. Squatting with knees *together*, put both hands on the floor to the left of the thighs. Inhale and move forward in a slightly diagonal direction, riding on the right arm, raising the feet from the floor. The legs should be kept together. Exhale as you come down, then practice on the other side.

(iv) Hair: teeth: eyes

Hair

The hair relies on the bloodstream for nourishment as does the skin of the face. It is thus affected by diet, sleep, the condition of the nerves and supplies of vital energy. It quickly reflects the state of the body, growing dull when health is poor. Serious illness, certain nervous disorders, even great anxiety or shock may turn it white or cause it to fall out.

Many people pay a great deal of attention to their hair but completely neglect the scalp, unless it draws attention by developing such unpleasant conditions as dandruff. They seem unaware that if scalp and hair roots do not receive enough blood, air and sunlight the hair itself will suffer, even to the extent of complete or partial baldness.

To supply scalp and roots with adequate blood, practise the Headstand (page 37); the Half-shoulderstand (page 35); the Head-to-Knee pose (page 70); and all forward stretching *asanas* (pages 36, 72). Also the forward-stretching movements on page 32 and exercises 1, 2, 17 and 22 on pages 28–31.

Other methods of stimulating circulation are occasional steambaths – wrapping hot towels round the head – and finger massage. The movement should be vigorous, the fingers 'dug in' and slightly bent to give greater pressure.

Brushing the hair, massaging the head in the open air, in sunlight, enables the scalp to breathe, to absorb some of the sun's vitamin D. Whenever possible the head should be dried out of doors after washing and excess moisture rubbed off briskly with a rough towel. The constant wearing of hats, caps, scarves, in and out of doors deprives the scalp of air, and felt hats in hot weather add sweat to this lack of air. Perhaps the worst offenders are women who go to bed with wet hair full of pins. If nothing worse, the result will be a greasy, clammy, unpleasantly-smelling head.

Extreme dryness, breaking, cracking, falling-out may come from a diet deficiency. A dessertspoon of oil every day will sometimes correct these faults in a matter of weeks, while certain fruit and vegetables containing silicon . . . apples, cucumbers, green peppers . . . will benefit and improve the hair.

To be beautiful, hair must be brushed every day. Brushing not only removes dust, polishes and disciplines, but also massages the scalp, stimulating circulation.

Regular washing is essential but this should not be done too frequently nor should strong soaps be used. A gentle, oil-based shampoo is harmless and a little lemon, vinegar or rosemary in the rinsing water makes the hair shine. If extremely dry, rub olive oil into the roots the night before washing.

Salt water should always be rinsed out after swimming. The dead cracked hair often seen on beaches in summer comes from combined salt water and over-exposure to strong sunlight.

Teeth

There is no substitute for a radiant, natural smile. Bad teeth have spoilt many beautiful faces and loss of teeth could add years to the appearance.

To keep the teeth healthy, blood circulation to gums and nerves must be maintained. Most of us forget the teeth have nerves until the dentist touches one in drilling; also that the teeth rely on the blood for nourishment, though we know that the system can be poisoned by dental decay.

All *asanas* and movements that direct blood to the head are recommended ... Headstand, Half-shoulderstand, Forward-stretching; also poses in which the chin is pressed to the chest ... Shoulderstand (page 50); Triangular pose (page 91); Cobra, with chin pressed in (page 61); Choking pose (page 92); the chinlock in *Uddiyana* (page 71). Practise the Pose of a Lion, and face and neck exercises on pages 29, 30 and 78.

Massage the gums with the fingers – towards the teeth – to increase the flow of blood and to discourage shrinking and recession. Chewing is also an excellent exercise for the gums (as well as facial muscles).

The teeth are affected by diet, which includes the water you drink. In certain parts of England many of the residents have false teeth – or go toothless – before they are out of their teens. For centuries lime was dug up for burning and the soil and water are now deficient in calcium. In such cases the diet could be supplemented by calcium and plenty of milk, also carrot juice.

Teeth and gums need Vitamins A and C. These are found – among other fruit and vegetables – in cucumbers, carrots, cabbage, celery, onions, tomatoes, parsley, pineapple, lemon and orange juice.*

Clean the teeth, if possible, after eating, particularly after sweet and sticky foods and always before bed. Upper teeth should be brushed downwards, lower teeth brushed in an upward movement. Brushing across encourages recession of gums. Be sure to brush well *between* the teeth where particles of food are often caught, causing decay.

If you are without a toothbrush, rinse out the mouth, swilling round the teeth. If they are stained by food – milkless tea ... black grapes – a little baking soda or lemon juice from time to time will clean them effectively.

An important measure not mentioned in traditional yoga literature but essential for western life, is to see the dentist regularly every six months, as a preventive measure. This will enable him to check any damage before it goes too far.

Eyes†

Children move their eyes constantly, whereas adults turn the whole head to see objects not directly in the line of vision.

We thus deprive the eyes of good and strengthening movement but this could be replaced by deliberate exercising. As well as the cycle on page 44 we could exercise the eyes in our everyday activities ... following moving objects, people in the streets, in the bus; at the

* Dandelion juice is highly recommended for teeth and gums.
† If the eye capillaries are weak – showing in bloodshot eyes – be careful about sending blood to the head. Examine the eyes after inverted poses and if there is any sign of extra redness, do not go on.

cinema or watching television letting them range over the whole screen as action changes.

When doing close work of any kind – sewing, typing, writing, etc. – it is a good idea to stop occasionally and change focus . . . lifting your eyes and looking at a distant point several times, then palming for a minute, putting the hands lightly over the closed eyes to shut out all light.

Since the eyes are dependent on the bloodstream they reflect the physical condition even more than hair and complexion. Everything shows in the eyes . . . wrong diet, lack of sleep, loss of vital energy, discontent, depression. Most of us abuse, overwork and neglect them, forgetting that their work never stops during waking hours; that they are constantly recording, watching, transmitting to the brain. We should give them all possible help through general care, diet and adequate provision of arterial blood.

The latter is supplied through all inverted poses or those sending blood to the face – as suggested for teeth and hair.

Diet should provide plenty of Vitamin A, so abundant in carrot juice and also found in apple, celery, cabbage, kale, parsley, pineapple and radishes.

Tired eyes should not be overstrained. Refresh them by bathing and a few minutes palming. Use either an eye bath or water as it runs from the tap. Water poured into a basin accumulates impurities which, splashed into the eyes, may irritate or even cause infection.

The best remedy for tired eyes is to stop work and go to bed early. It is surprising how often this simple remedy relieves strain and headaches.

Sun your eyes, with the *lids closed*. (*It is dangerous to look directly at the sun*). Sit facing the sun and slowly move the head from side to side, feeling the warmth of the rays on the lids.

Never read with strong sunlight on the book or with light in your eyes. At night, read only in a good light, trying to avoid bad print.

Dark glasses, except in conditions of extreme brightness, are a bad habit, particularly if worn indoors.

The following eye exercises are designed to improve and strengthen the power of focussing as well as developing strong muscles; therefore with each movement you should focus on a specific point. These exercises will not cure congenital deficiencies or serious diseases but they will maintain good optical health and delay the common symptoms of ageing – failing powers of quick focus and poor vision caused by muscular weakness.

Practice also Pose of a Lion (page 31), Facial exercises 15, 16 and 25, and *Savasana* (page 89).

Eye Exercises
1. Up, down; up, down; up, down, close.
2. Up, straight, down, straight; up, straight, down, straight, close.
3. Right, left; right, left; right, left, close.
4. Right, straight, left, straight; right, straight, left straight, close.
5. Looking up diagonally – right, down left; up right; down left; up right, down left; close.
6. Change – left up; right down, etc.

7. Circle eyes right round to the left. Circle round to the right.

8. Changing focus: look at the tip of nose, then into the distance. Repeat several times.

9. Look at tip of finger held about a foot from the face, then into the distance. Repeat several times.

10. Stare fixedly, trying to see more clearly without straining and without blinking.

11. Squeeze the eyelids together, then blink several times.

12. Massage eyelids by gently stroking them with first finger and thumb outwards from the nose, to the outer edges of the eyes.

13. Place the fingertips gently on the eyeballs (with eyes closed), and concentrate on breathing *prana* into the eyes. *Prana* may be directed to the eyes by breath and also, to a certain extent, through the fingertips.

14. Practise palming – placing the palms of the hands over the eyes to completely exclude the light.

Regular eye exercises – which could be done at any time, even lying in bed – brighten the eyes through stimulation of circulation and general toning-up. This brightness, together with expression and vitality, are more important than colour or setting. Some of the most striking, dynamic faces prove, on analysis, to have small eyes of no great physical beauty.

3

Beauty of Body

(i) General care

'Your best dress is the silk of your skin; your best armour is the armour of your muscles.'

To a yogi his body is a source of pride . . . not in the sense of empty vanity but as a reflection of his achievements. One of the main doctrines of hatha yoga is to preserve the *sameness* of the body right through life . . . to work against the changes that may come through physical ageing . . . alteration of weight, stiffening of the back and joints, failing digestion, flabbiness of muscles.

Most of these changes could be delayed, some brought to a standstill; in cases of premature ageing there could even be restoration . . . a refirming of flesh and muscles, a renewed suppleness of joints, a more youthful grace of movement. Results will vary according to the amount of concentration and practice the student is prepared to devote.

Grace, flexibility, posture. Movement is to the body what expression is to the face. As an unpleasant expression may negate fine features, the effect of a well-proportioned body is spoilt by bad posture and carriage, awkward movements, ugly walk, stiffness.

46

To be beautiful the body must be graceful and to be graceful it must be supple, relaxed, well co-ordinated.

In the Pacific Islands and the East one sometimes sees immensely fat women dancing with a grace that transcends physical ugliness. Sinuous arm movements, lightness of foot, 'boneless' flexibility and perfect co-ordination cancel out unsightly flesh. In the west, unfortunately, jerkiness, briskness are more common than sinuous gestures; the suggestion is of the drill hall rather than the dancing school. This may be due to the games we play, the lives we lead, but it is a fact that a graceful woman, a well co-ordinated man are so exceptional as to command immediate attention.

Ability to sit, stand, move with relaxed grace is one manifestation of yoga training. The constant emphasis on spine and joints ensures upright carriage and suppleness; breath control, training in relaxation correct *gauche*, jerky movements; while *asanas* will firm flesh and muscles, adjust weight – through exercise and effect on the glands – and keep the body in its best condition.

Proportions. Though certain exercises are said to increase height, specially in growing bodies, the bony structure of a fully developed adult will not be changed by exercise. The flesh, however, may be remoulded to improve the shape, through regular and serious practice. Figures, particularly in women, sometimes alter quite dramatically. Where the weight is normal there may be no difference shown on the scales, but a redistribution of fat takes place all over the body, bringing more harmonious proportions. (Correct weight with poor figure is not uncommon). In women, the most frequently noted improvement is redistribution of fat from hips to bust, but there are cases where boyish shapeless bodies have developed into gracefully curved, small-waisted feminine forms. Men develop in chest and shoulders, firming and slimming waistline and stomach.

Large stomachs are often caused less by fat than by flabby muscles. Regular exercise will tighten them and thus improve the figure.

Weight. No one can look their best if they are too fat, nor can they expect to really enjoy life. Apart from heart conditions, there are many disagreeable minor complaints aggravated by obesity – varicose veins and haemorrhoids among them.

If you are seriously overweight, restrict your diet. Cut out all the notorious fatteners . . . cakes, sweets, white bread and sugar, fried foods, TV snacks, coffee parties, soft drinks and alcohol. A water fast once a fortnight, a fruit or fruit-juice diet once a week will help keep the weight under control.

Water fasting

Choose a day when you will not be too busy and preferably when you can be alone. Eat no solid food all day, and drink only water. Conserve all energy, even keeping silent, if possible. Practise breathing cycles and go to bed very early. If the fasting is also for purification, an enema at the end of the day is suggested.

Fruit juice dieting

Follow the same procedure as for water fasting, substituting fruit juice.

Fruit diet

Eat only fruit during the day ... if much overweight this could be prolonged for 2 or 3 days. It should be the same kind of fruit – i.e. all citrus, all apples or all stone fruit. (Avoid acid fruits if your system is acid, and starchy fruits, like bananas, if you are constipated or have indigestion).

Fruit and nut diet

Eat only fruit and nuts.

Four-ingredients dieting

Eat fruits, nuts, vegetables and honey for 4 to 7 days.

It is necessary to exercise regularly every day during dieting, not only to reduce but to keep the body firm. Loss of weight often brings empty folds of skin or flabby tissues. Practise exercises for different parts of the body – selecting those you need from pages 57 to 79 and the following *asanas:* Shoulderstand (page 50); Headstand (page 37); Head-to-knee (page 70); Plough pose (page 70); Bow pose (page 60); Archer (page 69); Forward-stretching cycle (page 36, 72); Spinal twist (page 70); *Uddiyana* (page 71).

It is particularly important to practice the Shoulderstand daily for its effect on the thyroid gland. (The thyroid greatly influences weight). Where the problem is underweight, practise holding the Shoulderstand as long as comfortable, to stimulate the thyroid, then drinking warm goat's milk.

In case of extreme obesity, avoid the headstand till some weight is lost.

X *Shoulderstand or Candle Pose*

Lie down on your back with arms by the sides. Raise both legs, keeping them straight, up over the head. Support yourself with your hands. They should be holding the back, in the region of the shoulderblades, with elbows on the floor and arms forming a wedge to prop up the body. The body and legs, eventually, should be in one straight line, though this may take practice; but at all times the chin must be pressed firmly to the chest, against the thyroid gland. If this is not done the blood will go to the face and head, as in the Half-shoulderstand. The whole purpose of the pose is to drain arterial blood from legs and body and direct it to the thyroid. Retaining the pose – deeply inhaling and exhaling – allow time for this life-giving blood to stimulate, condition and regulate the gland. The effects are then transmitted to every gland in the body. Not only weight but vitality, mental attitude, ageing processes are involved. The mind should be concentrated on these benefits.

To complete the Shoulderstand, bring legs down over the head, keeping them straight, till the toes touch the floor, if possible. The hands should now be on the floor, roughly in line with the position of the hips when the body is lying flat. Hold this extended pose for a second or two, concentrating on the spine, then bend the knees, and slowly lower the legs back over the head and down to the floor. Completely relax.

General Care of the Body

Additional measures, apart from yoga *asanas* and exercises, are necessary to achieve or maintain physical beauty.

Care of the Skin

Ancient yoga instructions on skin care – particularly the skin of the body – include the following:

'Cut a lemon in two and sitting in comfortable cross-legged position rub and rub into elbows, so coarseness of the skin is eliminated. Wash off and rub in oil. Do the same with the knees and neck. Flatten half a lemon and rub into the skin under the chin in gentle up-and-down movements, thinking of the sameness of the skin all over the body; then rub in oil.'

Oil baths are described on page 26.

Air baths – lying in the shade, wearing a minimum of clothing – enable the skin to breathe freely.

In general, the rules given for care of facial skin apply to body skin . . . adequate protection, ventilation, absolute cleanliness. A bath or shower should be taken every day, if possible all the year round.

An important practice is to rub the body with a loofah, in the bath or shower, until the skin is stimulated to a gentle pink colour.

Particular care should be paid to the feet. Never allow corns to grow or ingrowing toe-nails to develop. Callouses on heels and soles of feet should be removed with pumice stone.

Diet

A great many problems of figure, face, complexion, general health, may be traced back to diet.

You may be eating too much meat, drinking too much alcohol, taking too much white sugar on food and in drinks. You may be going to too many tea parties, always picking between meals. The eating that accompanies any kind of visual entertainment – cinema, television, even theatre and ballet – destroys teeth, complexions and digestions, not to mention figures.

The body must have sugar for warmth and energy but this is available in honey, fruit and dried fruits. Honey, taken daily, soon destroys a craving for chocolates and cakes. Reduce meat consumption, if you are eating it more than once a day. Three or four times a week is ample, if fish, eggs, cheese are substituted on other days. The true yoga diet, of course, is vegetarian. Plenty of vegetables – not overcooked – salads, fresh fruit, fruit juice, nuts, water,* milk (if it agrees with you), yoghurt, buttermilk are all excellent foods, sustaining and healthgiving. White bread is no longer a necessity with so many excellent health breads now available, and like white sugar, it is best avoided.

It is important to eat at regular hours, allowing time to digest the meal. If you are unavoidably pressed, eat sparingly, cutting out heavy foods that tax the digestion. *Alcohol and tobacco.* These two poisons are completely antipathetic to yoga training. For all its convivial associations, alcohol taken to excess is a destroyer. An occasional drink, for social necessity, will do little harm, but if you suspect any tendency towards alcoholism in yourself, refuse it.

Smoking. The rule for yoga students, concerning tobacco, is: *Do not smoke under any circumstances.*

* Drink enough water every day.

Rest and relaxation. Sleep

Savasana, the yoga exercise in complete relaxation is described on page 89 and if practiced regularly the whole body and appearance will benefit. There are also other ways of relaxing . . . sitting in the sun or lying under the trees *doing nothing* – being idle with no sense of guilt or compulsion to rush about. It is a comment on our way of life that so many people must be taught to let go. One constantly hears the words, 'I can't relax'; but relax we must, if we are not to turn prematurely into old nervy men and women.

Try to practise *Savasana* in the middle of the day, which is thus divided into two parts. If you cannot lie down, sit with head drooped forward on the chest and the whole body and limbs completely relaxed.

Sleep. There are two main kinds of non-sleepers – those who cannot and those who do not. The former need help; the latter need more sense. It is one thing to stay up late for a good reason – theatre, travelling, an emergency – but staying up just to avoid going to bed is the worst kind of stupidity.

Those who wish to, but cannot, sleep, could improve their condition through deep breathing, relaxation, and the Pose of Tranquillity (Appendix). General practice so benefits health and nerves that better sleep usually results.

It may be necessary to adjust your sleeping conditions . . . make your bedroom darker or quieter, or if this is impossible, put cotton wool in the ears and a scarf or mask over the eyes. It is difficult to sleep in a stuffy room so be sure you have plenty of fresh air but do not lie in a draught. You may be sleeping with too many pillows, an uncomfortable or oversprung mattress; you may not be warm enough or supporting too many heavy bedclothes. You may have eaten too big a meal too soon before retiring, or have had a family row or be taken up with worry, unhappy or disagreeable thoughts. You may be overstimulated by work, a film, even a book. You may have just stayed up five minutes too long and lost the moment when you could have slept naturally.

Try to slow down before bedtime; go for a little walk, even a swim in summer. A warm bath often helps bring the relaxation needed for sleep, as does deep breathing by an open window, and *Savasana* after getting into bed.

If sleep does not come, do not panic. Lie quietly, breathing deeply, rhythmically, remembering that you are resting, relaxing muscles and nerves, and that if you master this art of relaxation you will have learnt to refresh yourself.

General exercise

Apart from yoga practice, get as much exercise as you can in your daily life. If you work in an office, shop, factory, walk in the city – if your shoes permit it – instead of taking buses. Garden, go for walks or swims at weekends. Housewives could get the maximum from housework by making exercises out of bending, stooping, moving about. If you live in an area where food is delivered, try walking to the shops a couple of times a week instead of taking the car. Judging by the number of housewives who flock to yoga classes this section of the community not only needs exercise but is honest enough to admit it.

Business men could, to advantage, use their cars less, even in the city. The usual excuse is lack of time; but when one adds up the time spent in traffic jams, waiting for lights to change, finding parking meters, it is likely to be more than that required to walk the distance, quite apart from the nervous energy expended.

Chronic unconscious tension

'Your hands lie open in the long fresh grass,
The finger-points look through like rosy blooms;
Your eyes smile peace.'

The tranquil mood of this poem is set by the image of the hands . . . calm, relaxed, serene, just as the mood of the body may be expressed by the hands, too often, alas, clenched in unconscious tension. Watch the hands in buses, in coffee shops. They are usually tightly closed, or clutching a book, paper, fork, umbrella, as though in desperation. Car drivers grasp steering wheels, whole body rigid; typists sit stiffly, frowning, typing in shattering, nerve-racking bursts; bodies, it seems, hurtle gracelessly through crowded streets as though competing in a never-to-be-won race. The tension is rarely released. At night these unhappy people sit with twisted legs and shoulders hunched, frowning at books or television screen; in bed, they lie screwed up in foetal postures, knees under chin, arms hugging chest, head thrust down into blankets. So it goes on night and day, living with tension until it becomes unconscious.

If you are one of these sufferers you could help yourself by learning and practising yoga breathing; by the regular

55

observance of *Savasana*, the Pose of Complete Rest which has restored peace to so many tense and harassed men and women. Mastery of these techniques soon brings a change in appearance, as well as in health; the eyes become brighter and softer, the movements more fluid and graceful and an air of repose is discernable. The feeling that life is really worth living, is not just a desperate rush, soon communicates itself to others and is reflected in your own face and personality.

(ii) *Exercises and asanas to improve the figure*

As we have already mentioned, it is possible to remould the human body, even in the case of fully-grown adults.

This is done by a number of slow movements, tensing and relaxing different groups of muscles, with the mind actively participating in the process. The student actually sculptures himself, part by part, as he practises the movements. In exercising the arms, for example, he should learn to project in his mind the image of his arms as he would like them to be; and the same with legs, shoulders, chest, waist, etc.

These slow movements could be dramatically effective with young bodies still in the process of development The system was known and used for hundreds of years in the Academies of Beauty referred to on page 81.

In many ways, modern isometric exercises follow the same principle

Each muscle is made of thousands of thread-like cells which may be slightly thickened by exercise. This is the basis of every body-building method, and when taken to extremes by enthusiasts results in the development of enormous muscles.

Yoga training does not give this over-development but, using the same principles, the student learns to bring the body to its best possible shape, and to retain it, firm and unchanged, all through life.

In cases of excess weight, the combination of wise diet and exercise could 'dry' up the body, slimming heavy hips, arms, stomach.

Before beginning practice, look carefully at your figure, assessing your worst points, not in a mood of despair but constructively, with the intention of improving them to the best of your ability. Regard your body as raw material to be formed as you wish; have faith that you will succeed and, should confidence flag or results come slowly, remember the hundreds who have not only improved their physical appearance but in the process developed will-power, determination, patience, achieving the sweetest of all victories . . . victory over self.

Exercises for chest and bust
1. Tensing and relaxing chest muscles. Imagine you are pulling yourself up on a rope. Raise the arms over the head and clenching the fists, pull down, tensing muscles of the chest, then relaxing when hands reach about chest level. Repeat four times. (For firming the bust).
2. Clasp the hands in front of the chest. Push with the right and resist with the left, tensing chest muscles, slowly *pushing*, against pressure, to the left, then pushing to the right. Repeat four times.
3. Hands in same position but this time fingers in an over-

locking grip. (With left palm facing up, curl fingers inward, then insert curled fingers of right hand, held palm downward). The movement now is *pulling* against resistance, pulling with the right hand, resisting with the left, moving across to the right, then to the left. Repeat four times.

4. With clenched fists together in front of the chest and elbows out. Pull the fists apart, as though against heavy resistance, tensing chest muscles. Pull back until shoulder-

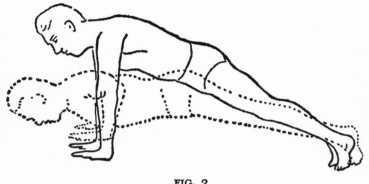

FIG. 2

blades are brought together, then relax and start again. Repeat four times.

5. Stretch arms forward with clenched fists facing inward. Keeping arms straight, slowly pull against resistance, opening the arms as wide as possible and at the same time leaning back from the waist. Relax, return to starting point and repeat four times.

6. Stretch arms forward with clenched fists, this time facing down, as though holding a bar. Slowly raise the arms, against resistance, above the head, keeping them

straight. Raise them as high as you can and slightly back over the head. Relax and repeat four times.

7. Lie flat on the back with arms by the side. Inhale, arch the spine, raising only the chest, then exhale and lower it. Repeat several times. Only chest must be raised ... shoulders, head and hips remain on floor.

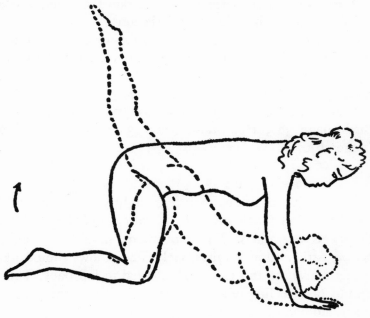

FIG. 3

8. *For men.*

With palms and toes on the floor, body stretched in 'press-up' position. Push yourself up, extending arms, then come down and press up again. Continue until pleasantly tired. (Fig. 2).

9. Practice same movement with the hands further apart.

10. Practice same movement with the hands closer together.

11. Practice same movement with hands further forward.

12. With palms and toes on the floor in press-up position, lower the body, raising right leg; come up, lowering leg; come down, raising left leg; come up, lowering leg.

These movements are too strenuous for women who should practice the following variation:

13. On your knees with palms in press-up position, touch floor with your chin, at the same time stretching right leg. Change sides and repeat. (Fig. 3).

Asanas for chest and bust

Practice also, Head of a Cow pose (page 34); Pose of a Bird (page 38); Headstand (page 37); Pose of a Hare (page 36).

Pose of a Camel (Plate 2)

In kneeling position, with legs slightly separated, arch the spine and reach behind till your hands are holding the heels or ankles. The movement should be one of *arching* rather than leaning back. The elbows should also be kept straight and the head allowed to fall back. There should be a feeling of stress in the muscles of chest, neck, waist, stomach and thighs.

Hold the pose as long as you can in comfort, inhaling and exhaling.

Pose of a Bow

Lie face downwards. Bend back the legs and take hold of the ankles. Inhale and pull on them, at the same time bringing up head and shoulders till the body forms a bow.

Pressure should be felt in the small of the back and the chest muscles tensed. Exhale and relax. Repeat once.

Pose of a Cobra (Plate 3)

Lie face down with palms on the floor, level with the shoulders. The chin and feet are on the floor, the toes flat, not pressed in. Inhale and arch the spine, raising head, shoulders, chest and putting pressure on the small of the back. Below the waist the body should be pressed to the floor. Exhale and come down. Repeat once more; then practice twice, pressing the chin against the chest.

Pose of a Peacock

A rather strenuous pose more popular with men than women, but excellent for developing firm chest muscles, and muscles of the back.

Kneel down with the palms on the floor, wrists turned so that fingers face towards the body. Stretch the legs out behind, keeping them together with toes touching the floor. Keeping the arms close together, bend the elbows and lean forward over them so that they press into the stomach, in the region of the liver. Inhale, and slowly move head and body further forward over the arms – elbows now pressing firmly into the stomach – until the feet begin to rise from the floor. Eventually body and legs are elevated with the whole weight taken on the hands.

Exercises for hips, buttocks and back

1. Lying on the back with knees bent and soles flat on the floor. Hands clasped behind neck. Inhale, raise the hips,

contracting buttock muscles, exhale and come down. Repeat four times.

2. In same position, inhale, raising hips and stretching one leg forward. Exhale and come down. Repeat on other side. Practice four times. (Fig. 4).

3. On back with hands by sides and legs stretched. Inhale and raise only the hips, arching back and keeping shoulders and heels on the floor. Exhale and come down. Repeat four times.

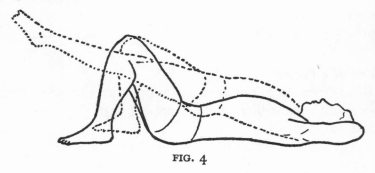

FIG. 4

4. On back with hands clasped behind head, draw the knees up to the stomach and massage hips by rocking from side to side in a slightly circular movement putting all weight on hips and buttocks.

5. Massage hips with knees bent and soles of feet on the floor, moving knees from side to side. Hands behind neck.

6. With legs stretched and hands behind neck, rock from side to side, slightly arching the back and putting all weight on the hips.

7. With arms at the sides. Rock over on to the right, then to the left, taking all weight on the hips.

8. Sit up with knees bent and apart, soles of feet together.

Put the hands on the ankles and rock from side to side, massaging the buttocks.

9. With hands on hips and legs stretched forward. Walk forward on the buttocks, pushing forward left leg, then right, then left, then right; then reverse and come backwards.

10. Sit up with arms folded on chest and both legs bent

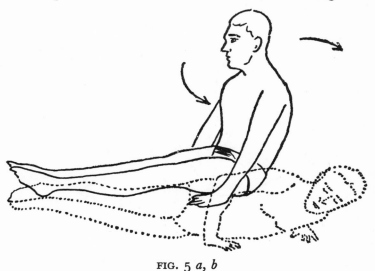

FIG. 5 *a, b*

to the left. Stretch legs out and up (about 45 degrees) in front, keeping them straight, then draw them in to the right side; stretch them up and forward again, then in to the left. Continue until tired, pivoting on the buttocks and trying not to fall over backwards.

All-over massage

Sit with the legs stretched forward. Put the palms on the

floor on the right side of the body and turn over on to the stomach, keeping the feet off the floor, so the weight is mainly on stomach and hands. (Fig. 5 *a*, *b*).

Continue rolling over to the right until you are sitting up again with a hand on each side of the body and legs stretched forward.

Swing the legs – keeping them straight – to the right, describing a semi-circle with the feet, pivoting on the buttocks. (Fig. 5 *b*, *c*).

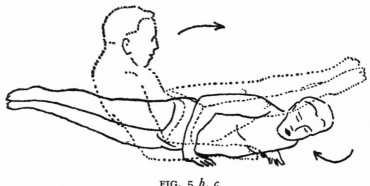

FIG. 5 *b*, *c*

Continue rolling over to the right on to stomach again, steadying yourself with your hands, if necessary, until you come back to starting position – sitting up with legs stretched.

Study the directions carefully and practice step by step. Then try to do them in a continuous movement of combined rolling and pivoting, until pleasantly tired.

This movement massages stomach, hips, buttocks and exercises the waistline. When done quickly enough, centrifugal force stimulates the circulation in the limbs, specially the feet; but as the blood is drawn off the solar plexus to a certain extent, the exercise should be followed by relaxation and recharging breaths.

It is much easier to practice on polished floor or fitted carpet. Rugs will slip with your movements.

Asanas for the hips, buttocks

Practice also Pose of an Archer (page 69); Spinal Twist (page 70); Pose of a Bow (page 60); Plough Pose (page 70); Head to Knee Pose (page 70); Angular Pose (page 74).

Sideways Swing

Sit with both legs bent to the right and arms linked over the head. Inhale and as you exhale swing several times over the bent legs. Repeat, then change sides and practice on the left side.

Variation of Sideways Swing

With the left leg stretched and right bent back at the side. Clasp the hands on top of the head; inhale; exhale and come slowly down over the bent leg, trying to touch the floor with the elbow. Come up and repeat on the other side.

Lotus Position

Sit on the floor with the legs stretched forward. Lift the left foot, bend the knee and set the foot in the right groin, then lift the right foot and bring it up into the left groin.

The Lotus or Buddha pose is not complicated but is often difficult for Europeans because of stiff hip joints.

Careful and persistent practice is the only way to master it, but there should be no forcing or straining.

Pose of a Fish

Lock the legs in the lotus position, lean back, arching the spine till the crown of the head rests on the floor. The elbows should be on the floor at the sides and the hands resting on the toes.

Hidden Padmasana

Lock the legs in the lotus position, then lie down on the stomach, with hands joining behind the back in position of prayer (fingers pointing upwards towards the head).

Exercises for the stomach

Strong abdominal muscles are not only aesthetically pleasing – acting as a corset to control the waistline – but are also very important to good health. They assist the digestive and elimative processes and contribute to a strong and healthy spine.

1. Standing straight, tense and relax stomach muscles several times. Pause, then repeat three or four times. Keep the fingers on the stomach and feel the muscles become hard, then grow soft.

2. Lie on the back with arms stretched over the head. Sit up, drawing knees up under chin and swinging arms forward and down with hands on the floor. Lie back, stretching the legs, arms stretched over head again. Keep continuous movement, swinging up and forward then back, till tired.

3. In the same position. Sit up, swinging arms to the left so palms rest on the floor; lie back with arms above head. Sit up, swinging arms to the right; lie back and relax. Repeat several times on each side. (Fig. 6).

4. Rowing. Sit up with knees bent and drawn up and hands reaching forward between the legs as far as the ankles. Imagine you are holding an oar. Lean back, at the same time stretching legs straight and pulling on the oar, bringing the fists up against the chest. The body should be at

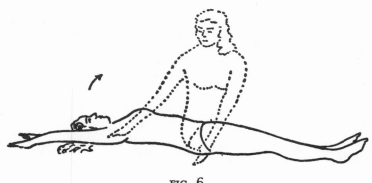

FIG. 6

about 30 degrees angle with the floor, all stress taken on stomach muscles. Then come forward again with arms between legs and knees drawn up; pull back again. Continue this rowing movement until pleasantly tired.

5. Lying on the back, draw the knees up against the stomach. Stretch the legs up (at right angles); slowly lower them to the floor, keeping them straight.

6. Lying on the back, hands on hips. Draw right leg up to stomach, then sit up – without help of hands – stretching the leg forward and up at 45 degrees angle to floor. Lie

down, bringing bent knee back to stomach. Repeat with left leg. Practice several times on each side.

7. In same position with hands at sides, draw both knees up, then sit up with legs stretched at 45 degrees. Knees back, lie down. (Fig. 7).

8. The same movement but this time stretch the arms out at the sides as you sit up and try to retain balance.

9. The same movement with hands clasped behind the neck.

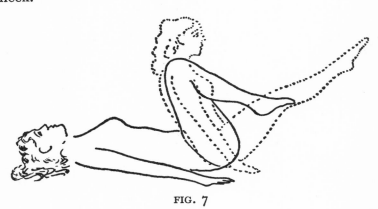

FIG. 7

10. With hands clasped behind the neck, draw knees up, stretch legs to 45 degrees angle, split them, bring them together again, bring knees back to body and lie down. During the stretching and splitting of the legs knees must not be bent.

11. Sit up with arms behind you and weight resting on the hands. Draw the right knee up and try to touch the right shoulder. Repeat several times; then practice with the left knee.

12. Half-reclining, legs stretched and weight taken on

elbows. With knees kept straight describe circles with both legs simultaneously raising them up, apart, down to starting position.

13. In the same position, circle the legs together, this time bending the knees, drawing them up to the stomach, stretching out and down, at the same time pivoting on hips and buttocks. (Fig. 8).

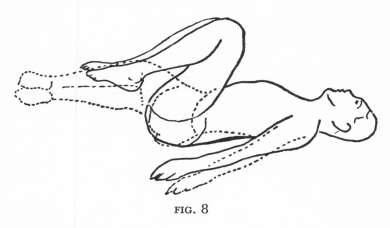

FIG. 8

Asanas for the stomach

Practice also: Shoulderstand (page 50); Half-shoulderstand (page 35); Pose of a Bow (page 60).

Pose of an Archer

Sit with the left leg stretched forward. Step over it with the right, putting the right foot flat on the floor, alongside the left knee. Inhale, exhale and lean forward, resting the *right* hand on the toes of the *left* foot and picking up the *right* foot with the left hand. Try to bring this foot up to the forehead till the big toe touches the spot between the eyebrows. The elbow should be held out and away from the body as you pull, the movement of an archer shooting an arrow. Come down, change sides and repeat.

Spinal Twist (Plate 4)

Sit cross-legged. Leaving the *left* leg in position, step right over it with the *right* leg, putting the right foot on the floor. Bend the *right* arm behind the back. Straighten the *left* arm in front, bring it over the bent knee (the *right* knee) and down, on the *right* side till the hand touches the floor. Keeping the arm straight and keeping it all the time on the *right* side of the knee, slide the hand gently along the floor till it reaches the *right* foot. (If you follow this step by step, carefully, you should not have difficulty working out the position). Inhale, exhale and twist the body from the waistline right round – to the right – until you are facing behind you. Return to starting point and practice on the other side.

Pose of a Plough (Variation)

Lying on the back, bring the legs right up and over the head till the toes rest on the floor. The arms should be linked loosely round the head and the knees kept straight; with the toes lying flat on the floor, gently slide the feet to and fro, coming as close to, then as far from the head as you can, stretching the spine. To complete the pose, bend the legs and bring them down as in the Shoulderstand.

Head-to-knee pose

Standing with the legs together and hands on the backs of the thighs, inhale, exhale and bend forward, drawing the stomach in and sliding the hands down the backs of the legs till they can hold the ankles. Press the head to the knees without bending the legs. Come up and repeat.

Uddiyana (Plate 5)

This difficult *asana* is essential to health and beauty and is listed as one of the most important of all yoga techniques. It provides deep internal massage for abdominal organs and brings mastery over semi-voluntary muscles. It not only stimulates digestion, cures constipation and certain menstrual irregularities but develops firm flat stomach muscles. It may be practised sitting or standing.

In standing position, separate the feet about 18 inches. Put the hands on the upper thighs, fingers pointing in towards each other. Inhale; completely exhale. Slightly bend the knees, lean forward, putting weight on the heels of the hands and at the same time press the chin to the chest and try to draw the stomach right *in* and *back*, in a slightly upward diagonal movement. Imagine you are trying to pull it back against the spine, at the same time raising the diaphragm, making a deep cave under the ribs. Retain the contraction for a couple of seconds, then relax. You must exhale all air from the lungs before contracting the stomach.

When you have mastered the contraction, try to contract and relax more quickly as a continuous flapping movement, in, out, in, out. It is not easy, but leaning forward, slightly arching the back and taking the weight on the hands will give more control over abdominal muscles.

Uddiyana should never be practised on a full stomach –

(at least 3 hours after a meal) – and it is not advisable for women *during* menstruation. The best time is early in the morning while the stomach is empty. Practice until you can make up to 25 consecutive contractions.

Forward stretching cycle. (See also page 36). All movements to be practised on both sides.

Arch Gesture

Sit with the right leg stretched and the left leg bent with the knee on the floor and the sole of the foot pressed against the right inner thigh. Inhale, exhale and lean forward, trying to grasp the right foot with the hands, pressing the head to the right knee. Do not bend that knee. Come up, repeat; then change sides and practice twice more.

Variation 1

With right leg stretched and left foot up in right groin, in half-lotus position.

Variation 2

With both legs crossed. Inhale, hold the toes with arms outside the knees, exhale, coming down to touch the forehead on the floor.

Exercises for the waistline

Practice also the exercises on page 32 for bringing blood to the face.

1. With feet apart and elbows out at the sides; put fists together in front of chest. Pull apart, as though against resistance, at the same time turning the body to right,

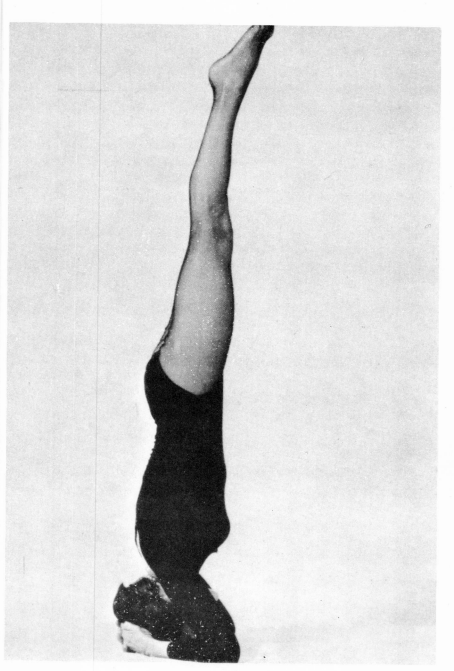

Plate 1: Headstand

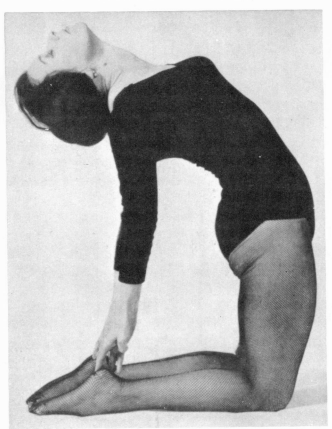

Plate 2:
Pose of a Camel

Plate 3:
Cobra pose

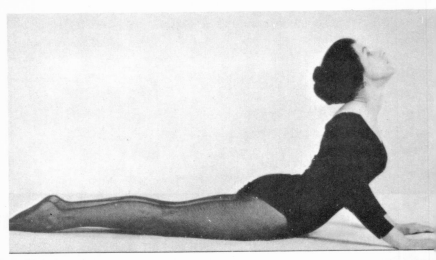

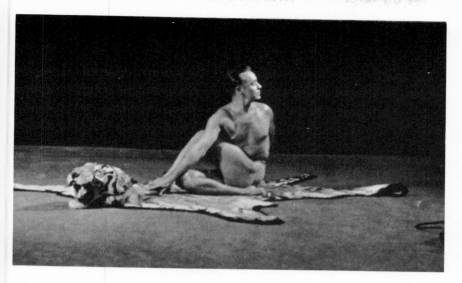

Plate 4: Spinal Twist

Plate 5: *Uddiyana*

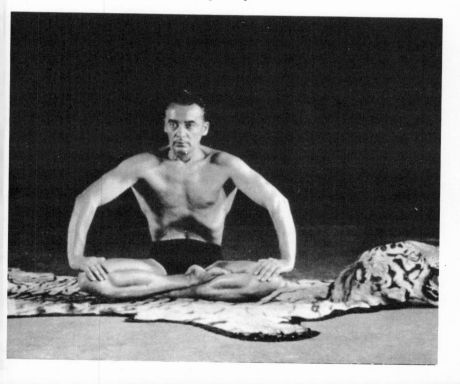

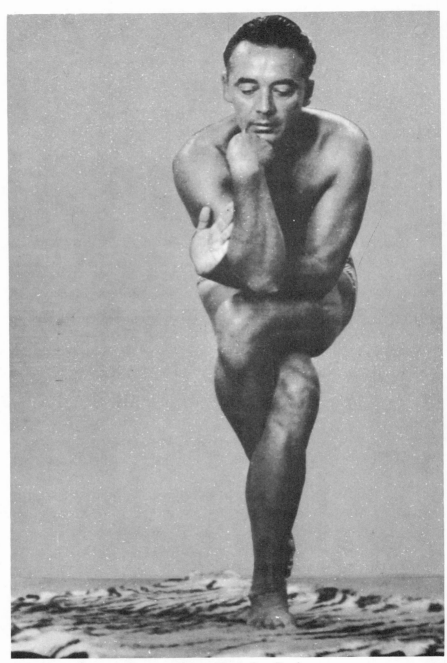

Plate 6: Pose of an Eagle

from waistline, keeping feet flat on the floor. Come forward and repeat to the left. Practice several times on each side, making sure that all twisting movement is in the waist.

2. With feet apart and arms stretched at the sides. Come down on the right side, touching the floor with the right hand. You may bend the right knee as you bend and the left arm should be straight up in the air. Repeat on other side.

3. With feet apart and hands on backs of thighs. Inhale, exhale and bend forward, running hands down backs of legs to take hold of ankles and pressing the head first to the right knee, then to the left.

4. With feet together, clasp hands over the head, arms stretched. Bend right over to the left, then to the right, bending at waistline.

5. In same position, twist, from the waistline to the right, then to the left.

6. With feet together, imagine you are lifting a heavy weight with your left hand, raising it up under the armpit. At the same time the right arm and shoulder go down. Come up and raise imaginary weight with right hand, letting left arm and shoulder go down. The movement should be felt in the waist muscles.

7. The same movement with the feet apart, which enables the descending arm to go down further, giving more exercise to waist muscles.

8. Stretch both arms up and out to the right, bending from waist. Relax. Stretch out to the left. Relax.

Asanas for the waist

Practice also Sideways swing and variation (page 65);

Spinal twist (page 70); all forward-stretching (page 36, 72); Cobra (page 61). Also Exercises on page 32.

Angular Pose

Sit with the knees bent and drawn up. Take hold of the big toes and slowly stretch the legs out and up till they are fully extended and at an angle of 45 degrees with the floor. You are balancing on the buttocks with the legs wide apart. Hold the pose, then relax.

Vajroli-mudra

Sit with knees drawn up and hands at the sides, palms on floor. Inhale, stretch the legs up and out, at 45 degrees to the floor, keeping them together. Hold; then exhale and come down.

Exercises for the legs

1. Standing with feet together, come up on to ball of the foot, then on to the toes – in two movements. Come down and repeat several times, tensing muscles at the back of the legs.
2. With hands on the hips, practice stationary walking, not taking the feet from the floor but fully exercising the leg muscles.
3. With hands on thighs, practice a half-squatting consecutive movement in 1–2–3–up rhythm. Repeat several times.
4. With hands on hips, rise up on toes, then come down into full squatting position. Repeat 3–4 times.
5. With arms stretched forward, come down into squatting

position, then try to sit back on the flat of the feet, tensing muscles and tendons at back of ankles and calves.

6. Standing on right foot, raise the left with knee bent and swing the calf back and forth several times. Repeat on other side.

7. On right foot, raise left leg as above but instead of swinging back and forth move leg to the side – keeping knee bent – then forward, to side, then forward. Repeat on other side.

8. Standing with feet apart and hands on hips. Keep soles flat on the floor and bring the knees in together, slowly, till they touch, then apart, together, apart, tensing thigh muscles.

Asanas for the Thighs

Practice also Pose of a Camel (page 60); Pose of a Bow (page 60); Cobra (page 61); Head to Knee (page 70); Lotus position (page 65); Fish pose (page 66); Hidden *padmasana* (page 66); Eagle pose (page 77).

Supine Pelvic

Sit back on the heels, arch the spine and try to come back over the feet till the crown of the head is on the floor. The hands are held in position of prayer. In the early stages you may help yourself back with hands and elbows.

Pose of a Star

Sit with the knees apart and the soles of the feet one against the other. The hands rest on the ankles. Inhale, exhale, leaning forward, taking hold of the feet with the hands and trying to press the forehead to the toes. The elbows should come down to touch the floor outside the legs. This is very strenuous and should not be over-practised.

Splits

Sit with legs as far apart as possible. Inhale, exhale and come forward, trying to put a hand on the toes of each foot and pressing the head to the floor between the legs. The knees must not be bent.

Pose of a Locust

Lying on the stomach with the face turned to one side. Stiffen the arms and put them under the thighs with the fists clenched. (Turn them so the thumbs rest on the floor). Inhale, and with a quick movement raise both legs, keeping them straight; exhale and come down. Keep the face on the floor all the time.

Asanas for calves and ankles

Practice also forward stretching cycles. All following balancing poses to be practised on right and left side.

Pose of a Tree

Stand on the right foot. Bend the left leg back and holding the ankle with the left hand, bring the heel against the buttocks. Keep the knees together. Arch the back, look up, and raise the right arm. Hold the balance as long as comfortable; come down and repeat on the other side.

Variation of Tree pose

Stand on the right foot. Lift the left foot at the ankle and bring it up into the right groin, in the half-lotus position. Retain it there while joining the palms together over the head. Repeat on other side.

Pose of an Eagle (Plate 6)

Stand on the left foot. Slightly bend the knee and wind the right leg round, from the front, hooking the right foot round the left calf. *The position is identical with sitting on a stool with legs twisted round each other.* Lean forward and twist the arms in the same way, leaning the elbows on the upper knee and the chin on the back of the hand. Repeat on other side.

Squatting balance (i)

In a squatting position but with knees together. Support yourself with the right hand on the floor, take hold of the left foot with the left hand and stretch it right out in front – keeping knees together. When you feel you can hold the balance, take the right hand from the floor and rest it on the right knee. Hold it as long as comfortable; then change sides and repeat.

Squatting balance (ii)

Squat on the floor with knees slightly apart. Cross the left calf over the right thigh and try to maintain balance, taking all the weight on the right foot.

1. The hands should be in position of prayer.
2. Held out at the sides.
3. Palms joined over the head.

Repeat, balancing on the other leg.

For the arms

Practice also all Raised poses: Bird, page 38; Raven, page 39; Peacock, page 61; Head of a Cow, page 34; Pose of a Camel, page 60.

Exercises for the arms

1. With feet together and arms stretched out at sides, clench the fists and bend the elbows, flexing the biceps. Relax. Repeat 5–6 times.
2. Starting with finger-tips on shoulders, move the arms out at the sides in an undulating movement as though pushing against the air. Continue till arms are tired.
3. Clench fists and bring the arms up from the sides and forward to about chest level, tensing arm muscles, then relaxing. Repeat 5–6 times.
4. The same movement but with a 'Scooping' movement. When fists are about at waist level turn them inward, downward and outward, twisting at the wrists, so that biceps and triceps are exercised. Lower arms and repeat. Practice several times.

For the Neck

Practice also Pose of a Camel (page 60); Supine Pelvic (page 75); Headstand (page 37); Shoulderstand (page 50); Half-shoulderstand (page 35); Pose of a Fish (page 66).

Neck exercises

1. Sitting with legs crossed: raise head up, then lower it; up; down; up; down.
2. Turn head from side to side, repeating four or five times.

3. Slanting the head from left to right four or five times.

4. Raise the head, then let it drop forward, quite limply, three or four times.

5. With hands clasped at back of neck, press down and forward and at the same time resist with the neck, creating a feeling of tension in the muscles. (This is an important exercise for good posture and for preventing Dowager's Hump).

6. Push the chin out, then draw it back; out; back; out; back. (For double chin).

7. Slowly circle the head right round to the right, slowly and in a very relaxed way; then repeat to the left.

8. Briskly tap neck and under chin with fingertips to stimulate circulation.

4

Inner Beauty

'My first encounter with my teacher was unforgettable. As he came in, the rather-badly lit room of his *ashram* actually seemed to grow brighter.

'I saw a man about forty, of medium height, with supple, graceful movements and firm fresh skin. His features were not classical, even regular, but his calm face literally radiated light.

'Later, seeing him daily, I tried to analyse what made him so beautiful. The general impression was of extreme kindness, of deep penetrating understanding, untainted by any inharmonious thought. It was as though I had met my elder brother after years of wandering in a strange world. I felt good, secure, *warm* with him. This was more than physical beauty. Inner beauty shone through him, and this, once seen, is never forgotten.'

This is Michael Volin's description of meeting his Tibetan-Chinese teacher, who was then over seventy. Others have described similar experiences. A famous writer once said his most impressive war memory was the face of a nurse bending over him as he recovered consciousness, a woman – never seen again – who personified goodness. Some of us have perhaps seen a great musician, physically unprepossessing, transformed as he played; an ugly actress radiating light and grace through the words she interprets; insignificant listeners exalted by music or poetry; plain women become great beauties through the expression of noble thoughts or emotions.

What is inner beauty? It is the individual's inner quality ... yoga calls it a 'balance of forces of soul'. It is tranquillity; peace; a 'quiet mind'; goodness, spiritual enlightenment; the 'pilgrim soul'; true understanding of the beauty round us, love of nature; compassion; noble humility; simplicity; above all, love of humanity ... acceptance of everyone as a new and wonderful experience.

We are drawn towards these qualities when we encounter them, just as we are repulsed by such negative traits as malice, hatred, envy, discontent.

The literature of the classical period of Chinese culture describes Academies of Beauty, where a trained teacher from Tibet worked on selected boys and girls, moulding them physically into beautiful animated statues, and developing their inner beauty by teaching them music, the art of writing poetry with the lightest strokes of the brush on silk, and the art of love. These practices have been continued in Japan, while, in the west, until the last generation, such accomplishments as singing, playing an instrument, painting, dancing were part of a young lady's education. The custom, though it perhaps degenerated into banality, was inspired by a desire to cultivate the inner being, to express something other than materialistic thoughts.

Yoga training in the cultivation of inner beauty may, in some cases, amount to a re-education, a complete change of attitude in the inner self. There are few qualifications needed, apart from the desire to succeed, though ability to surrender self, become utterly absorbed, identified with a thought, object or experience is necessary, and far more valuable than cleverness.

Traditional methods or 'exercises' for inner beauty are usually suggested by the teacher.

1. *Love of nature*

'All rivers flow in my veins; all mountains are locked in my heart; all clouds are reflected in my eyes. I am the earth and sky – all and everything.'

Unity with nature purifies and develops mind and soul.

Make every effort to spend some time daily – if only a few minutes – in the open. Make yourself receptive to the life round you . . . trying to understand esoterically why and how flowers are opening, birds singing, insects flying, willow trees swaying . . . as it were *participating* through your absorption. These quiet hours in the open air not only benefit physical appearance but contribute to inner strength and tranquillity.

This practice leads to love of the elements.

2. *Love of the elements*

To love, enjoy, fully experience every mood of the elements . . . sunshine, heat, cold, rain, gentle breeze, blue sky, storm clouds . . . to become completely receptive and aware of them is to increase the joy of living in this world. They provide energy that enriches the soul – a fact recognized by true creative artists, many of whom instinctively turn to the elements – even the fiercest tempests – to recharge their forces of soul.

Development of spiritual qualities
Music

Music is the purest and most universal means of communication, of expressing the divine aspect of the human spirit.

Mantra yoga – the yoga of sound vibrations – teaches that through complete surrender to sound one becomes sound itself. *Ohm Breath* is an ancient exercise leading to this identification.

3. Sit with legs crossed, or lie down in the pose of *Savasana*. Establish deep and rhythmical breath; then change the rhythm – after deep and slow inhalation, retain the breath long enough to concentrate on the sound of '*Ohm*', silently evoking it within you. Exhale. Inhale again, and again retain breath, hearing *Ohm*. Exhale. Repeat this until your whole being has become one vibrating sound . . . beautiful and mighty as the pulse of the universe.

4. Master this exercise, then learn to 'become' music. Listen alone, (or with a completely attuned companion). Lie fully relaxed on the floor, in *Savasana*, deeply and rhythmically breathing. Do not try to *understand* the music . . . accept it with your whole body . . . receive it fully, without reservation; let it flow through you, trying to merge with it, dissolving self into sound.

5. *Painting; sculpture*

As with nature and music, surrender self in contemplation of sculpture, painting, exquisite works of art. Identify yourself with their loveliness and in doing so absorb and retain their essence.

This book is written for *karma yogis* – followers of yoga

who are householders, married or single, living a life of action in a busy world. If they choose, they could find means of developing inner beauty everywhere, thus turning daily life and surroundings into spiritual experiences.

This is the path of action; but there are also other methods of cultivating inner beauty. The exercises given below are practised in the cross-legged position, with steady rhythmical breath established . . . six heartbeats to inhale, six to exhale.

6. *Releasing of Inner Light*

Although this exercise has also a physical aspect in that it releases facial tension, it is of the highest spiritual significance.

In yoga, Inner Light means the soul, the spark of God, of divinity. The more clearly it shines through the physical shell, the greater the beauty; but the stresses and difficulties of living too often obscure its pure light. We must learn to reveal it, to discard over-shadowing tensions as a germinating seed discards its outer case; as the grub discards its chrysalis . . . breaking through into radiance.

In cross-legged pose, with breath established, turn the whole mind to the systematic relaxation of every part of the face, eliminating all tension; *giving way* completely; offering no resistance to the beauty within that seeks to show itself.

7. In a more difficult exercise known as *Concentration on Inner Light*, the mind is focussed upon the immortal nature of the soul. This helps to overcome fear of death.

8. *Concentration on Inner Sound*

In the exercises *Ohm Breath* and *Music* we touched on identification with sound. This exercise goes further. Yoga teaches that Inner Sound . . . 'a faint tinkling bell' . . . is not only the origin of all music but of all beauty; the seed of all inspiration.

Starting with cross-legged pose and breath established, try to detach yourself from external sounds, withdrawing into yourself, dulling your physical powers of hearing. At the same time, listen inwardly, with full concentration. After faithful practice the serious student will eventually become aware of this mysterious 'music of the soul'.

9. *Attunement to Universal Goodness*

In this exercise, as in those on nature and music, self is discarded. The whole being is made receptive to the quality of goodness. Concentrating upon thoughts of courage, compassion, generosity, upon the simple kindnesses and noble aspirations we see or read of every day, identify yourself, tune yourself to this mood of universal benevolence, sharing and experiencing its peace and happiness.

10. *Object of love and devotion*

'Her pale face was enlightened by the beauty of a woman in love', wrote Ivan Bunin. Countless other writers have expressed the same thought, for love is the greatest beautifier of the human face. This may be seen in many different ways, in every country, every walk of life . . . the expression of a mother watching a child; exchange of glances between lovers; the adoration of a simple peasant kneeling in a village church. For some the greatest love may be for ideals ... for causes ... for humanity; for others, for God alone.

Whatever you love most should be held in your mind, all thoughts directed upon it. Practising deep and rhythmical breathing, surrender self, letting the power of love flow through and illuminate you.

This exercise might be compared, in a way, to *samadhi*, in which the yogi's soul is united with the soul of the universe. *Samadhi* is the supreme identification and its ineffable joy completely transforms the face of one who achieves it. Though it may sometimes come involuntarily, for most it requires long training and for the ordinary man or woman of the west remains an unknown experience. But the cultivation of inner beauty lies within the reach of all who wish not only to improve appearance but to enrich their lives.

Appendix

Breathing, Relaxing, Sleep

How to breathe correctly

Breathing is the basis of physical yoga and the method must be mastered before *asanas* are practised. It is a deep complete breath which fills and empties the lungs with each inhalation-exhalation. Standing with hands on the waistline, breathe in through the nose, at the same time expanding the stomach. This movement lowers the diaphragm and allows the bottom of the lungs to fill with air. Continue the inhalation, feeling the middle ribs expand, then the upper ribs. The lungs are now full. To exhale, breathe out through the nose, drawing the stomach in. This raises the diaphragm and begins to empty the lungs. The breathing is slow and rhythmical. It is, actually, in three stages, as described above but as practised becomes one continuous movement. There should be no lifting of the shoulders, typical of shallow chest breathing, and all inhalation-exhalation is done through the nose, unless otherwise stated.

Breathing cycles

To recharge energy. (Inhaling through the *nose*, exhaling through the *mouth*).

1. Stand with feet together, by an open window or in the open air if possible, arms by sides. Inhale, retain the

breath, clench the fists and tense every muscle in the body, holding breath and tension. Then exhale and relax.

2. With feet together, arms by sides. Inhale and raise arms forward, clenching fists as though holding iron bar. Retain breath and tension; exhale and relax.

3. Feet together and arms by sides. Inhale, raising arms forward. Clench fists and pull the arms vigorously back against the shoulders, forward, back, forward, back, then exhale and relax.

4. Feet together, arms by sides. Inhale and raise arms forward; retaining breath, move arms apart, to sides, then forward again; to sides; forward; to sides; forward. Exhale and relax.

5. Feet together and arms by sides. Inhale and swing both arms up over the head, down, up, down, up, down. Exhale and relax.

Cleansing breath

With feet apart, inhale, bringing arms up from the sides till they are over the head; then throw the body forward from the waist, exhaling vigorously. The arms fall forward and head and arms dangle limply as you bend. Repeat three times. Always finish breathing cycles with a Cleansing Breath to get rid of any stale air left in the lungs.

During this Cycle – which replenishes energy in the body – the actual recharging is done during exhalation. With inhalation the energy or *prana* is taken into the lungs; with exhalation, only stale air is breathed out; the *prana* is directed either through the whole body – or to any part that needs revitalizing – or to the solar plexus where it is stored.* Direction is done by the *mind*. Recharging exercises lose their power if practised without full concentration.

Pacifying cycle
To soothe the nerves. Advisable before going to bed, if a bad sleeper. (Inhaling and exhaling through the *nose*).
There are nine deep peaceful slow breaths in this cycle. Practise with closed eyes.
1. Inhale, slowly bring arms up and forward in a circular movement, crossing in front of the body, then up over the head and down at the sides as you exhale. Repeat four times.
2. Inhale with arms coming up at the sides to join over the head; exhale bringing arms down. Repeat three times.
3. Inhale bringing arms forward and up over the head; exhale coming down. Repeat twice. All through the cycle concentrate on the thought of peace.

For relaxation. Savasana – Pose of Complete Rest
It you can, darken the room as much as possible, then lie down on the floor, on your back. Shut your eyes. Your arms should be by your sides, your legs together, but not rigid.
1. *Relaxing the muscles*. With your mind completely withdrawn from other subjects and from your surroundings,

* The solar plexus is the reservoir of *prana* or vital energy.

concentrate on your muscles. Starting with the joints in the toes, try to relax every group right up through the body . . . feet, ankles, calves, knees, thighs, hips, stomach, waist, small of back, chest, shoulders, arms, hands, neck, lower jaw, tongue, eyes, forehead. Hands should lie lifelessly, jaw sagged down, tongue limp, eyes rolled back under the lids, habitual frown wiped out. Eventually, after practice, it is possible to relax every muscle in the body. It must be done slowly and with no sense of 'forcing' which will set up tension. If you find it hard to start, take a deep breath and tense the whole body, then relax. Do this a couple of times.

2. *Withdrawal of nervous energy.* This is harder since it involves relaxing the nerves, the emptying of tension from the thousands of nervous channels. Imagine a great slow wave is rolling over you, washing away all the inner tension, the feeling of being driven and pent-up. Let it all go; let everything go; let yourself sink; try to feel so limp and lifeless that you could not lift a finger. Imagine you are sinking down, down, through the floor.

3. *Recharging through breath.* Begin to inhale and exhale the full deep abdominal yoga breath, letting the stomach come out as you breathe in, and fall back as you breathe out. The rate of the breathing is far slower than normal – about six heart beats to each inhalation, six to each exhalation – and this slowing down is imperative, for it is the medium by which you assist relaxation. Slowing down breath eventually slows down the whole body and helps the nerves to release tension. *At the same time concentrate on recharging, sending prana through the nadis or nervous channels.*

4. *Detaching the mind*. Try to send your mind right away into some peaceful and beautiful place that you know or have created in your imagination ... it does not matter where, so long as it brings thoughts of happiness and tranquillity. The traditional yoga mental retreat or *ashram* is a lovely garden. With all the power of mind and will, imagine you really are in this retreat, secure from all usual worries, responsibilities, irritations. For a few minutes escape completely. You may need to use great willpower if you have pressing worries on your mind but you *must try*. The ability to forget for a few minutes, the power to escape, is the great secret of being able to carry on.

In the very last stage, and the hardest of all, switch off the thoughts and pictures and try to keep the mind blank. Only practice and slowing down of the breath will bring this state of real peace. It will help if you keep your eyes rolled back under the closed lids.

A few minutes of *Savasana* properly practised will entirely refresh you.

To improve sleep. Pose of Tranquillity (Triangular Pose)

Lying on the floor on your back, stretch your arms over your head. Raise your legs as though for the Candle or Shoulderstand. Keeping both legs and arms *straight*, raise the arms and support the legs with the hands, forming a triangle with body and limbs. This is achieved by balance and may need some practice. You should feel perfectly comfortable and secure with the weight taken on the back of head, neck and top of shoulders. To complete the pose, split the knees, bring them down over the head into the

Choking Pose. Take hold of the backs of the knees and press the bent legs to the floor. This puts pressure on the thyroid gland. Then let go, slowly lower legs and arms and relax.

Regular practice of this *asana* has so improved sleep in many cases that sleeping pills have been discarded.